Off the Beaten Path: Non-Traditional Careers for Medical Professionals

Dr Ashe Coxon & Dr Amandeep Hansra

ISBN: 978-1-7638831-2-3

DEDICATION

To the doctors who have reached out in moments of struggle,
and to those who have responded with kindness, wisdom, and support -
thank you for reminding us of the power of connection.

To the early supporters who gave us the courage to begin -
your encouragement lit the way.

And to our families,
whose unwavering support has sustained us every step of the journey -
we are deeply grateful.

CONTENTS

1	Introduction	Pg 1
2	Some important questions	Pg 3
3	Figuring out your why	Pg 11
4	Boards & Committees	Pg 21
5	Digital Health	Pg 23
6	Insurance Sector	Pg 26
7	Management Consultancy	Pg 29
8	Medical Advisory	Pg 32
9	Medical Media	Pg 35
10	Medical Writing	Pg 38
11	Pharmaceutical Industry	Pg 40
12	Portfolio Careers	Pg 42
13	Public Health	Pg 44
14	Regulatory & Policy	Pg 46
15	Research	Pg 49
16	Start Ups & Entrepreneurship	Pg 53
17	Venture Capitals	Pg 55
18	Others	Pg 57
19	Maximising Your Skills	Pg 58
20	Job Searching	Pg 61
21	Linkedin	Pg 63
22	Final Words	Pg 65

ACKNOWLEDGMENTS

Creating the content for this book required the collaboration between Dr Amandeep Hansra (Creative Careers in Medicine) and Dr Ashe Coxon (Medical Career Planning) who have > 20 years combined experience in assisting doctors in their careers. It has been a deeply meaningful journey, and it would not have been possible without the encouragement, insight, and support of many people.

To the doctors who have trusted us with their stories, allowed us to walk alongside them in moments of uncertainty, and shared in the hope of something more, thank you. Your honesty and courage continue to inspire us.

To the countless doctors who have extended their hand to a colleague with advice, a listening ear, or simply the reassurance that they're not alone. Your kindness, support and generosity with your precious time does not go unnoticed, so thank you.

To the Creative Careers in Medicine dream team: Dr Elise Putt, Sophie Turner, Dr Jason Lam, Dr Cheryl Martin, and Adam Rushford, thank you for your thoughtful book edits, feedback, and unwavering support throughout this process. Your input has helped shape this book into something we are truly proud of.

To the early champions of our work, thank you for your belief in the vision and for giving us the push we needed to begin. Your support gave us momentum when it mattered most.

To our families for the endless patience, love, and sacrifices behind the scenes thank you for grounding us and making space for this work to grow. We are deeply grateful for your unwavering presence.

Finally, to the broader community of doctors exploring new paths, questioning the status quo, and redefining what a fulfilling medical life looks like we see you. We wrote this book for you.

Ashe and Amandeep

INTRODUCTION

Medicine isn't a one-way street with a prescribed destination, instead it's a vast landscape of possibilities, both clinical and non-clinical. Yet, for many doctors, finding the right path can feel overwhelming, especially when career indecision, lengthy training programs, uncertainty in acceptance onto competitive training programs, job insecurity and burnout loom large. With so many options to choose from, and a growing desire among clinicians to expand their skills and explore roles beyond the bedside it's no wonder that navigating your next steps can feel daunting. This guide is here to be your compass, helping you uncover the diverse, rewarding opportunities in the non-clinical world and empowering you to craft a fulfilling career that aligns with your interests, values, and aspirations.

This book is designed to help medical professionals explore career options beyond traditional clinical roles and includes industry exploration tips, strengths and transferable skills identification.

The inspiration to write this book stemmed from a collaboration between Dr Ashe Coxon and Dr Amandeep Hansra, who have spent a combined 20 years educating doctors, medical students and other health practitioners on non-clinical and non-traditional options for healthcare workers.

Book Overview

This book covers several key topics essential for healthcare professionals considering a move into non-clinical roles, including:

- Key considerations before embarking on a non-clinical career.
- An exploration of common non-clinical career options available to medical professionals.
- A breakdown of what these roles involve, and the skills required to succeed in them.
- How to begin your job search in the non-clinical field.
- Guidance on identifying transferable skills and how to effectively showcase your expertise when transitioning to a non-clinical role.

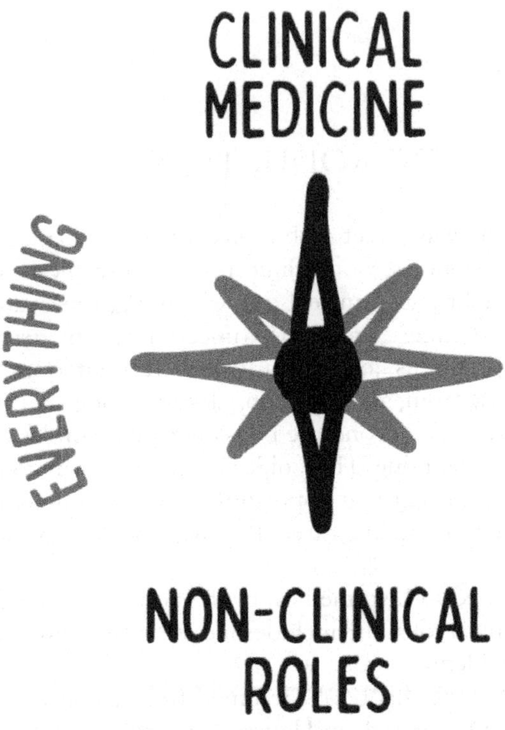
CLINICAL
MEDICINE
EVERYTHING
INBETWEEN
NON-CLINICAL
ROLES

SOME IMPORTANT QUESTIONS

Before we delve into the different non-clinical medical careers, it's essential to take a moment to reflect on a few key questions. These are important considerations that can influence your decision-making, particularly if you're transitioning from a clinical to a non-clinical role. Whether you're currently practicing medicine or have already stepped away from clinical work, these questions will help you navigate this transition thoughtfully.

For many doctors, the excitement of exploring non-clinical opportunities doesn't necessarily mean they are ready to leave clinical medicine entirely. Some may still want to maintain a connection to clinical practice, while others are certain that clinical medicine is not the right fit for them. Both paths are completely valid, but it's essential to be aware of certain factors that could affect your employability and job security in a non-clinical role.

If you've already decided that non-clinical medicine is the right direction for you, it's crucial to consider **four key aspects**. There are many factors that will personally impact your own career decision making, and it is important that you also address those and not just the ones below, but if you can find answers to these four big questions then you have had a fantastic beginning to your career journey!

The following section will guide you through how to find the answers to these four important questions;

- Do you want to **obtain** General Registration?
- Do you want to **maintain** your medical registration?
- Do you want to work with patients?
- Why do you want to move into non-clinical medicine?

Question #1: Do You Want to Obtain General Registration?

If you have already obtained general registration, you might ask yourself if you wish to maintain it. However, for who haven't yet obtained general registration, such as medical students, interns, or international medical graduates who haven't yet completed the necessary steps, this question becomes more pressing.

General registration, which is governed by the Medical Board of Australia, is typically a period of supervised practice. Successfully completing this process allows for more flexibility in your career, especially if you wish to maintain the option to work in clinical roles such as locuming, career medical officer (CMO) work, or any role that requires direct patient care. It's also beneficial if you pursue non-clinical roles that might still expect or benefit from general registration, such as positions in public health or medical advisory roles.

For many, maintaining general registration acts as a safety net. Should a non-clinical role not work out, having the option to return to clinical practice offers a sense of security. It can also bolster your confidence when exploring new opportunities, knowing that clinical work is more than likely available (As long as you maintain your mandatory requirements such as CPD etc).

If general registration isn't possible or right for you, it's important to discuss your options with a career counsellor, coach, a trusted friend or family member, colleagues or a mentor. In some cases, there may be ways to navigate the registration process with certain accommodations.

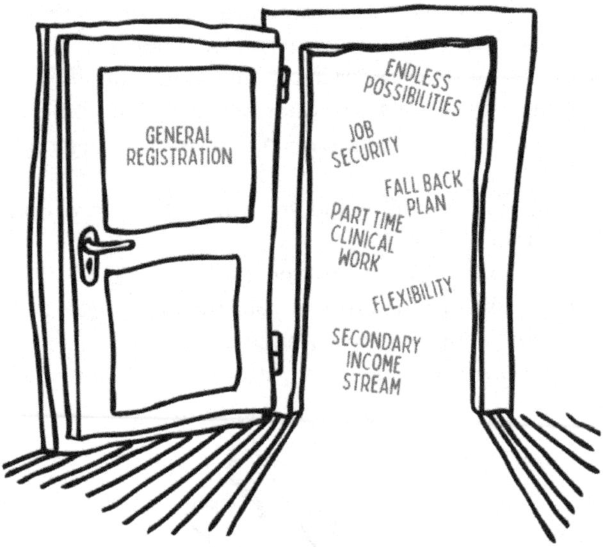

Question 2: Do You Want to Stay Registered as a Doctor?

Maintaining your medical registration is different from obtaining general registration. While general registration involves supervised practice, staying registered means you continue to meet the obligations set by the Medical Board of Australia, which requires ongoing engagement in medical work, such as a minimum of 152 hours per year plus CPD requirements (as of 2025. Before making any big career decisions please always be aware of your specific/ individual registration requirements)

Maintaining your registration is generally easier than allowing it to lapse and attempting to re-register later. Re-registration often involves a return to supervised practice, which can be challenging after a prolonged absence from clinical work. Before making any decisions, consult the Medical Board's guidelines on registration and the different types available.

https://www.medicalboard.gov.au

The page below provides some guidance on non-clinical work and your registration obligations.

https://www.medicalboard.gov.au/codes-guidelines-policies/faq/faq-recency-of-practice.aspx

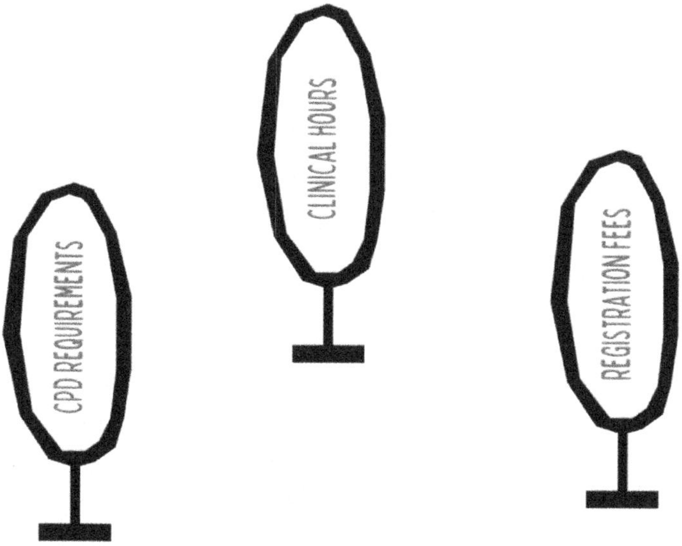

Question 3: Do You Want to Work with Patients?

This question may seem out of place in a book on non-clinical careers, but it's crucial to determine if you enjoy patient interactions. Even in non-fellowship medical options, there are roles that still involve patient care in varying capacities, such as clinical trials investigators, CMOs, or surgical assistants.

Other non-clinical roles, such as those in public health or medical administration, do not involve direct patient care but require medical fellowship. There may potentially be CMO roles, or unaccredited registrar roles in the areas, but the usual standard for employment is as a specialist in the field (With Fellowship). In these fields, you're not engaging with patients directly, but the work still impacts patient care on a broader scale.

Lastly, there are purely non-clinical roles where you may not need fellowship. However, some fields may consider a fellowship desirable, even if not required. For instance, if you're close to completing a fellowship, it may be worth finishing, as it could enhance your employability, especially in niche areas such as medical advisory roles within pharmaceutical companies. It is always a good idea to enquire about the expectations before making any big career decisions (E.g. Speaking with a connection in the industry if interest to see if a fellowship or registration is essential, desirable or not required at all.

Below is a useful exercise which will be useful to determine;

a. Whether you want to continue patient care, non-clinically or clinically; and

b. Why you may or may not wish to work with patients directly.

The insights from this exercise will be very useful to help you create your future career goals, options and trajectory.

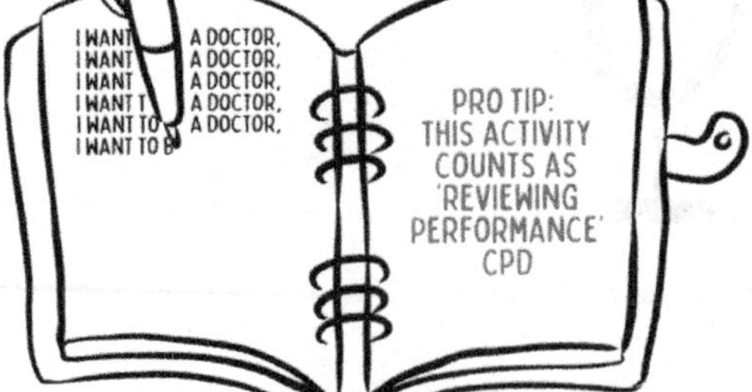

Exercise: Understanding Your Relationship with Patient Care

Purpose: To reflect on your experiences and feelings about working with patients to determine how much direct patient involvement you want in your future career.

Instructions: Grab a pen and paper, or open a document, and work through the following steps. Take your time to reflect deeply and be as honest as possible in your responses.

Step 1: Reflect on Your Positive Experiences

Think about your past experiences working with patients. Write down:

1. Memorable Moments: What is one moment with a patient that brought you joy or fulfillment?
2. Why It Stands Out: What specifically made this moment meaningful? Was it the human connection, solving a complex problem, or making a tangible difference, or anything else?
3. Strengths in Action: What strengths or skills did you use in that moment (e.g., communication, empathy, problem-solving)?

Step 2: Explore Challenges or Frustrations

Reflect on aspects of patient care that feel draining or unfulfilling. Answer these questions:

1. Challenging Moments: What is one experience with a patient that left you feeling stressed, frustrated, or unhappy?
2. Why It Stands Out: What about this situation was difficult for you? Was it emotional labour, time constraints, or feeling powerless to help? Is there anything else you can identify?
3. Patterns: Do similar challenges appear often in your work?

Step 3: Connect Your Reflections to Career Goals

Based on your answers above:

1. What do you enjoy most about working with patients? Are these elements you'd want to keep in your career?
2. What aspects of patient care would you prefer to avoid? Why?
3. Do you feel a sense of purpose or satisfaction from having a direct impact on patient lives? Or do you feel you could make an equally meaningful impact in a different, non-patient-facing role?

Step 4: Imagine Your Ideal Workday

Close your eyes and visualise your ideal workday in the future.

1. Are you interacting with patients directly, indirectly (e.g., through systems or policies), or not at all?
2. What kind of impact are you having on healthcare or society?
3. How does this vision align with what you wrote in Steps 1 and 2?

Step 5: Summarise Your Insights

Write a summary of your thoughts in response to this question:

- Based on this exercise, do I want to continue working directly with patients, indirectly support the patient journey, or shift entirely away from patient care? Why?

Question # 4: Why Do You Want to Move to Non-Clinical Medicine?

Understanding your motivations for transitioning to non-clinical work is key. Are you feeling burnt out? Is your current work environment toxic or unfulfilling? Or do you simply want to explore new ways to apply your skills?

Identifying your reasons can help clarify whether non-clinical medicine is the right choice or if changes within your current clinical environment could improve your situation. Some doctors pursue non-clinical careers because they feel their skills are underutilised in their current roles and they are eager to explore new opportunities.

Whatever your reasons, it's important to take the time to reflect on them. If any concerns arise during this process, consider reaching out to a career counsellor for support.

Take the time to reflect on these four questions as you begin this journey. Understanding where you stand on these key issues will provide a solid foundation for your transition into non-clinical medicine. If any uncertainties or questions arise along the way, don't hesitate to seek guidance from a mentor or career counsellor.

Exercise: Discovering Your "Why" for Non-Clinical Medicine

Purpose: To explore the reasons behind your interest in non-clinical medicine and determine whether this transition aligns with your goals and values.

Instructions: Take some time to thoughtfully answer the questions below. Write down your responses so you can revisit and reflect on them throughout your decision-making journey.

Step 1: Identify Your Current Feelings About Clinical Medicine

Reflect on your current clinical role. Ask yourself:

1. What aspects of my clinical work do I enjoy the most?
2. What aspects of my clinical work leave me feeling drained, stressed, or unfulfilled?
3. Am I experiencing burnout or dissatisfaction? If so, what do I think is causing these feelings (e.g., workload, environment, lack of growth)?

Step 2: Explore Your Motivations for Transitioning

Consider why you're drawn to non-clinical medicine. Answer these questions:

1. What excites me about exploring non-clinical work?
2. Do I feel my current skills are underutilised? If so, in what ways?
3. Am I seeking a better work-life balance, new challenges, or opportunities for growth?

Step 3: Consider the Possibility of Change Within Clinical Medicine

Sometimes dissatisfaction stems from the environment or specific circumstances rather than the work itself. Reflect on the following:

1. Could changes in my current clinical role (e.g., workplace, specialty, hours) improve my satisfaction?
2. Have I explored all options to make clinical medicine more fulfilling?
3. Would I feel regret or relief if I stepped away from direct patient care?

Step 4: Clarify Your Goals and Vision

Use your answers from Steps 1-3 to define your goals. Write down:

1. What do I hope to gain from transitioning to non-clinical medicine?
2. What impact do I want to have in the healthcare field or beyond?
3. How does pursuing non-clinical medicine align with my long-term aspirations and values?

Step 5: Take Action

If you're still unsure, consider:

1. Speaking to doctors who have transitioned to non-clinical roles for insights and inspiration.
2. Working with a mentor or career counsellor to explore your motivations and plan your next steps.
3. Revisiting your responses periodically to ensure your decisions align with your evolving goals and needs.

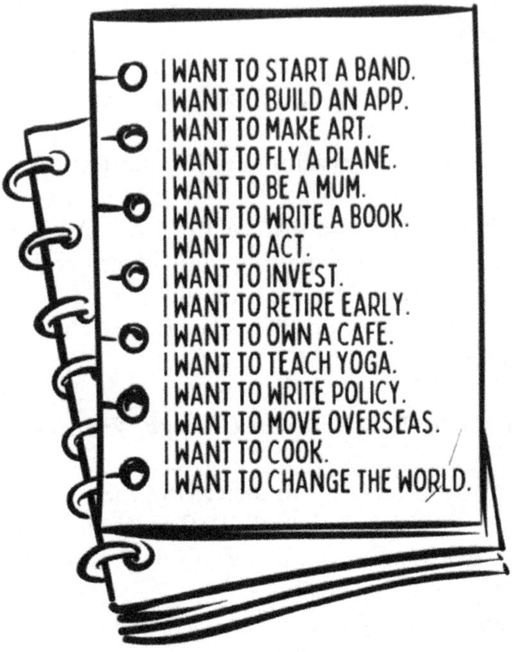
I WANT TO START A BAND.
I WANT TO BUILD AN APP.
I WANT TO MAKE ART.
I WANT TO FLY A PLANE.
I WANT TO BE A MUM.
I WANT TO WRITE A BOOK.
I WANT TO ACT.
I WANT TO INVEST.
I WANT TO RETIRE EARLY.
I WANT TO OWN A CAFE.
I WANT TO TEACH YOGA.
I WANT TO WRITE POLICY.
I WANT TO MOVE OVERSEAS.
I WANT TO COOK.
I WANT TO CHANGE THE WORLD.

FIGURING OUT YOUR WHY

Tailoring the Journey: Understanding Your Stage and Career Path

This book has been designed for a diverse audience, ranging from medical students to experienced doctors contemplating retirement. Some of you may already be working in non-clinical medicine, while others are considering transitioning from clinical roles. There will be people with and without medical registration, people who have never worked clinically, and those who are currently practicing. No matter where you are in your career, this book will offer valuable insights. It's structured to help you explore non-clinical career opportunities, irrespective of your experience or career stage.

However, it's crucial to recognise which stage of contemplation you're in regarding a shift to non-clinical medicine. You may recall learning about the stages of change during medical school: pre-contemplation, contemplation, preparation, action, and maintenance. When considering moving from a clinical field to a non-clinical one, or even skipping clinical training altogether, it's essential to identify where you fall within this model.

Most of you reading this book will likely be in the **contemplation** stage and curious about non-clinical careers, wondering what they involve, and questioning whether such a path is right for you. This stage often coincides with feelings of confusion or dissatisfaction in your current role. These feelings are common among doctors, and it's important to understand that career dissatisfaction doesn't necessarily mean a permanent shift away from your current path is needed. But if you're in that contemplative phase and are experiencing dissatisfaction, you should take some time to reflect on what drives career fulfillment for you.

What Brings Career Satisfaction?

It is useful to analyse what brings career satisfaction to you, and there are usually many, many influencing factors that may bring career satisfaction that are also usually very specific to your individual circumstances (e.g. work hours, family opinions, drive and ambition, financial etc). As there are so many factors that can contribute to career decision-making, many people find themselves confused and uncertain as to what they should prioritise.

For this reason, it can be useful to use a framework that helps analyse career satisfaction based on several key factors. Medical Career Planning has developed a career decision-making framework, the 'INSPIRE' framework (Interests, Non-Negotiables, Skills & Strengths, Personality Traits, Individual Core Values) and working through this framework can assist greatly in career clarity.

1. **Interests**
2. **Non-Negotiables**
3. **Skills & Strengths**
4. **Personality**
5. **Individual Core Values**
6. **Reality**
7. **External**

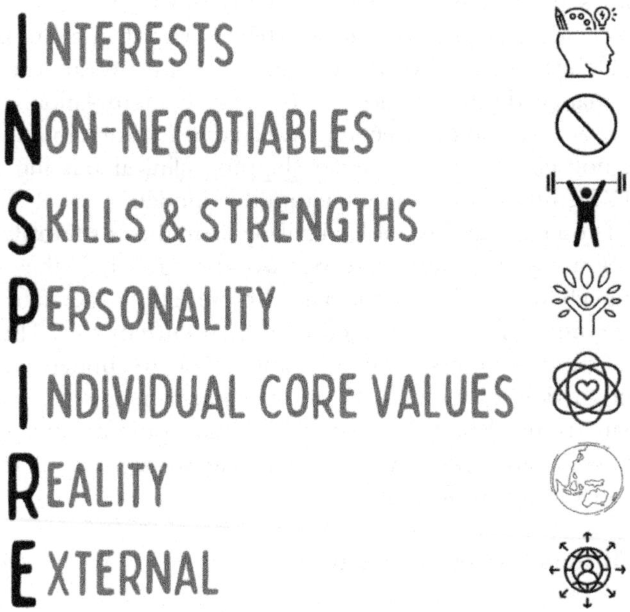

Each of these elements plays a key role in shaping whether you feel fulfilled in your current or potential career. Let's break them down:

Interests

When you're feeling unsatisfied in your career, start by reflecting on your interests. What excites you? What do you enjoy within and outside of medicine? Over time, doctors can lose sight of their interests as they become engrossed in their training and work. It's essential to revisit what truly captures your attention whether that's problem-solving, analysing data, or even hobbies like puzzles or collecting. Once you know what excites you, consider how these interests can align with a clinical or non-clinical career. Think both about your medical interests and your intellectual and personal interests outside of medicine.

ACTIVITY: Write down five medical interests (don't think too hard, just write down the first five things that come to mind) and then be specific with the definition

1. ______________________
2. ______________________
3. ______________________
4. ______________________
5. ______________________

For example:

1. Teaching or mentoring medical students and junior doctors. = Education
2. Performing procedural work such as endoscopy or minor surgeries = Procedure (Tip - If procedures is an interest of yours, further elaborate and define. E.g. - Short, non-operative procedures; Lifesaving procedures; Long procedures; Using fine motor skills; using gross motor skills etc)
3. Explaining complex medical terms in an easily understood manner = Translation
4. Tangible outcomes
5. Problem Solving

ACTIVITY: Now write down five non-medical interests, then analyse why you enjoy them and could you replicate that interest in medical fields.

1. Lego building. Why: Enjoyment from repetitive activities that have a process or set of instructions to follow (This may align with careers like anaesthetics, radiology, pathology, public health? Careers that involve

attention to detail and protocols for some of the career)
2. Creating jewellery. Why: Freedom to problem solve and create own solutions (?? Career that allows problem solving as core component)
3. Sport. Why: Enjoy outdoors (? Sports medicine. Nonclinical career that involves being outside)
4. Etc____________________________
5. Etc____________________________

Skills & Strengths

Identifying your skills and strengths is equally crucial. Later in this book, we'll dive deeper into how to recognise your abilities and translate them into the non-clinical world. For now, reflect on what you excel at and how those skills may fit into a new role. Showing future employers how your clinical skills transfer to a non-clinical environment is key.

ACTIVITY: Write down five skills (don't think too hard, just write down the first five things that come to mind).

1. ____________________________
2. ____________________________
3. ____________________________
4. ____________________________
5. ____________________________

Here are some examples of common skills within medicine.

Technical skills

- Rational prescribing
- Fine detail procedural skills
- Fast paced decision making
- Suturing/ wound care, plastering
- IVC insertion and venesection
- Resuscitation efforts E.g. CPR, intubation
- Interpretation of pathology tests/ findings
- Fast speed of work in times of need
- Data analysis

Problem solving and critical thinking skills

- Analytical thinking
- Creative thinking
- Solution-oriented thinking
- Ability to ask questions well and use different questioning techniques if required
- Open-mindedness

- Critical analysis

<u>Communication skills</u> (It is important to be **<u>specific</u>** here!)
Some examples.

- Verbal communication
- Non-verbal communication
- Written communication
- Body language
- Clarity of language
- Ability to give feedback
- Active listening

<u>Interpersonal skills</u>

- Empathy
- Dependability
- Patience
- Compassion
- Sensitivity
- Flexibility
- Conflict resolution
- Teamwork
    - Ability to work within a team
    - Ability to lead a team
    - Multidisciplinary teamwork
    - Collaborator

<u>Attention to detail</u>

- Observation
- Organisation
- Focus
- Time management
- Delegation
- Attentiveness

<u>Others</u>:

- Professionalism,
- Learnability
- Resilience
- Agility
- Creativity
- Leadership/ Management
- Negotiation

Personality

While personality traits shouldn't dictate your career choice, they can influence what environments or tasks you naturally gravitate toward. Understanding your preferences and any potential blind spots can help you navigate your career path. If you'd like to explore your personality more thoroughly, a Myers-Briggs Personality Course is available on www.medicalcareerplanning.com.au (QR code below. 50% discount code for book owners. Use the code BOOK).

Core Values

Your values, what's fundamentally important to you, must align with your career for you to feel fulfilled. Many people are not aware of their individual core values and how these impact our career satisfaction, so a useful exercise is to consider what one's values are and whether work is satisfying these. This can be done by completing the below exercise and then comparing your core values to your current career plans and identifying if they are similar or different. You can then be aware of what values may not be being met (If any) and then choose how to approach this.

Another exercise is to compare careers in which you may be shortlisting (E.g. Emergency Medicine Vs General Practice Vs Medical Advisory) and compare which may be most aligned with your values.

Remember, that having a career that suits your core values is just one component of career satisfaction, however for many people it is one of the most important considerations.

Now is a good time to begin thinking about what you truly value, whether it's autonomy, work-life balance, innovation, or making a social impact.

Below is a following exercise that will assist to identify your core values.

ACTIVITY: Choose 5 of the below values that you think lead to *personal satisfaction and motivation.*

- Solving problems
- Communicating
- Teamwork

- Ethics - work that is closely aligned with what you think is important
- Knowledge - challenges me to continuously improve and apply my understanding and intellectual capacity
- Independence - able to work when I want and how I want
- Creativity - able to use my creative and innovative ideas and/or artistic talents
- Research - find out new information and facts
- Help others
- Public contact
- Solitude - working by myself or in small group
- Make things
- Attention to detail
- Stability - offers me ongoing work according to my needs
- Change & variety - enables me to do different things quite often

Choose 5 of the below values that you think lead to feeling *awarded and appreciated.*

- Security - I want to limit financial and employment risk
- Influence people - persuade others and change their behaviour
- Lead and manage others
- Location - is in a location that appeals to me
- Intellectual status
- Make decisions
- Attractive workplace
- Recognition - gives me credit for my work and efforts
- Status - is in a career that is highly regarded in the community, and I hold a position that is highly regarded in the industry
- High income - the ability to generate above average income
- Competition - enables me to compete my abilities against others and rewards winning
- Ability to earn profit - enables me to increase my income through generating sales or investing
- Supervision
- Advancement - lots of opportunity for rapid promotion
- Negotiate - the scope to close deals and create opportunities

Choose 5 of the below values that you think lead to a *preferred lifestyle.*

- Leisure
- Community - ability to work with and help large numbers of people
- Excitement - is in a career that offers me new experiences and opportunities

- Help society - is a career that makes a difference in the world
- Work with others
- Fast pace - a job with lots of action requiring rapid decisions
- Adventure
- Work inside
- Friendships - work that allows me to develop close relationships
- Time & freedom - gives me the time to pursue the things I like
- Travel
- Work physically - using my body as well as my mind
- Work under pressure
- Work outdoors - not be caught up behind a desk or inside
- Learning - the opportunity for continuous learning & growth

You should now have a list of 15 'most important values' from the above list. Can you narrow this list of 15 down even further to identify your **top three core values.** If you have more or less that 3, that is completely fine, but make sure you try to limit it to not more than 6. For this exercise to be impactful you need to know what is most important to you.

Feel free to get creative - you don't have to stick to the words above! You can add in any values that you feel are important to you but may not be on the list.

Jot them down below:

1. ____________
2. ____________
3. ____________

Non-Negotiables

Next, it is essential to identify your non-negotiables. These are the conditions that you simply cannot compromise on, whether they involve financial stability, hours, geographic location, or specific job obligations. Knowing your non-negotiables helps you avoid situations where you feel trapped or unfulfilled. For those moving into non-clinical roles, understanding these factors before making a switch is vital.

Jot down some non-negotiables here;

1. ____________
2. ____________
3. ____________

Reality (and Expectation)

Reality and Expectation encourage you to reflect on the practicalities of your career and align them with what you hope to achieve. Reality encompasses the tangible aspects of your work, such as job availability, work-life balance, financial stability, return-to-service obligations, scholarships, or moratoriums that may affect your career choices. Expectation, on the other hand, examines what you envision for your career—your aspirations, goals, and desired lifestyle. When these two areas are misaligned, dissatisfaction can arise. By honestly evaluating the gap between reality and expectation, you can identify actionable steps to bridge them or redefine your goals to better match what is achievable. This alignment is crucial for sustainable career fulfillment.

External

External factors refer to the influences outside of your control that can shape your career decisions or contribute to career indecision. These might include family responsibilities, geographical location, economic conditions, job market trends, and societal expectations. External factors can also encompass organisational culture, workplace dynamics, and support networks. While these elements may feel overwhelming or restrictive at times, acknowledging their impact allows you to approach career planning with greater clarity and realism. By factoring in these external considerations, you can make informed decisions that balance your professional aspirations with the external realities of your life.

Reflect and Act

If you have ever experienced career dissatisfaction, think about the INSPIRE elements: interests, non-negotiables, skills & strengths, personality, individual core values, reality and external. Which of these areas is lacking in your current role? By pinpointing the missing factor, you can create an action plan to address it.

Once you've clarified your needs, you can shift into the **action** stage of change, where you start making real adjustments to your career. You might decide to pursue a non-clinical career or make changes in your current role to bring it more in line with your needs. Either way, keep these elements in mind as you navigate your path forward.

Whenever you feel that dissatisfaction creeping in, use the INSPIRE framework to assess the situation, determine what can be changed, and take action to create a career that truly satisfies you.

Next bits!

Now you have reflected on these important questions, we will dive into learning all about the non-clinical options!

Throughout the next sections you will be given information on different roles, industries and careers, and some tips of resources, websites or organisations that may assist. The list is not exhaustive, and there will be many other useful resources and websites not mentioned (And perhaps not even yet created by the time this book is printed!) so please ensure that you also do some of your own research.

Creative Careers in Medicine (CCIM) and Medical Career Planning (MCP) are resources that are referred to regularly, so here is the contact information for these organisations.

Creative Careers in Medicine (CCIM)

To join CCIM visit the website at https://creativecareersinmedicine.com
Or use the QR code here

Join CCIM Facebook page here: QR code

Follow CCIM on Instagram at @creativecareersinmed
Follow CIM on LinkedIn at https://au.linkedin.com/company/creative-careers-in-medicine

Medical Career Planning

To book an appointment or access online courses, webinars, blogs and events for Medical Career Planning visit the website at https://www.medicalcareerplanning.com.au/ or follow the QR code below

Join MCP Facebook page at https://www.facebook.com/medicalcareerplanning.com.au
Follow MCP on Instagram at @medical_career_planning
Follow MCP on LinkedIn at linkedin.com/company/medical-career-planning

BOARDS & COMMITTEES

Boards play a critical role in the governance and strategic direction of companies and organisations. Board members are appointed as either executive or non-executive directors. Executive directors typically hold senior roles within the organisation and are actively involved in its daily operations. Non-executive directors, on the other hand, are not employees of the company; they participate primarily in board meetings and may engage in specific tasks outside these sessions, including sitting on other board subcommittees.

The board is collectively responsible for overseeing the organisation's performance and ensuring it complies with regulatory and compliance frameworks. This often involves working closely with the CEO and senior executive team to guide the organisation's strategy and performance. Board members must work collaboratively to govern, direct, and monitor the organisation's progress.

The time commitment for board directors can vary widely, depending on the size and type of the organisation. Board meetings might occur monthly, quarterly, or even less frequently, and many boards have subcommittees that meet separately. Directors are expected to participate in these meetings and complete a significant amount of pre-reading of board materials in preparation.

In some cases, board members receive no compensation, especially in not-for-profit or volunteer boards, where they may only be reimbursed for expenses, such as travel. However, in for-profit organisations, directors are often compensated, though the amount can vary greatly. At the highest level, such as in ASX-listed companies, board members can be paid substantially, and in larger organisations, this role may even require a full-time commitment.

To be effective, board members need a range of skills. Doctors, for example, bring valuable expertise to the table, especially if they have non-clinical experience. Essential skills for any board director include strategic thinking, a high-level vision, and a solid understanding of financial matters, even if they are not experts in the field. Risk management, regulatory compliance, stakeholder engagement, and digital transformation awareness are increasingly important as well. Different boards prioritise specific expertise, depending on their focus, such as healthcare, aged care, or other sectors.

Doctors, with their problem-solving capabilities, strategic thinking, and risk management experience (especially in clinical governance) are well positioned to serve on boards. Leadership roles, experience on advisory boards, and qualifications like the Company Directors Course (Australian Institute of Company Directors) can further enhance a doctor's suitability for these positions. When considering joining a board, it's essential to perform due diligence to understand the organisation's financial health and legal responsibilities. Many doctors, early in their board career, begin by serving on not-for-profit boards or charity boards, gaining valuable experience before moving into paid positions on larger boards.

For those looking to explore board roles further, opportunities can be found through executive search firms, organisations like AICD, and networks like Women on Boards. Developing a tailored CV and application for non-clinical roles is crucial, as is preparing for interviews focused on leadership, governance, and strategic oversight, rather than clinical skills.

If you're keen to build a career in boards and governance, starting with advisory committees or subcommittees in your clinical setting is an excellent way to gain experience. Remember that board roles require a significant time commitment, including preparation and out-of-session work. Be mindful of balancing these roles with your clinical responsibilities to ensure you can engage fully and effectively in your governance duties.

DIGITAL HEALTH

Introduction

Digital Health is transforming the way healthcare is delivered, managed, and experienced. As technology continues to reshape and influence medicine, it is creating a wide range of non-clinical career opportunities for healthcare professionals. This chapter explores the dynamic and fast-evolving field of digital health and health informatics, examining emerging roles and innovative career pathways. It also provides practical guidance for those considering a full or partial transition into this area.

What is Digital Health?

Digital health encompasses a wide range of roles that leverage technology to enhance healthcare delivery, improve data management, and introduce innovative, technology-based models of care. But what does this mean in practice? It involves working with emerging technologies such as robotics, artificial intelligence (AI), chatbots, genomics, high-tech devices, or digital therapeutics. These technologies are poised to transform healthcare by enabling solutions such as prescribing apps instead of medications, virtual care models, telehealth, e-prescribing, electronic health records (EHRs) with AI based Clinical Decision Support algorithms, wearables, and Internet of Things (IoT) devices like in-home sensors.

These innovations not only enhance patient care but also address the growing workforce shortage, especially as we face an ageing population with increasing chronic disease. The ability to harness technology will be vital to meeting future healthcare needs.

The Role of AI in Medicine

AI is particularly noteworthy in its potential to revolutionise various specialties. Fields like dermatology, radiology, and pathology are already benefiting from AI-driven diagnostic tools, and the application of AI is expanding across all aspects of medicine. One prominent example is the use of natural language processing (NLP) to streamline administrative tasks. For instance, clinicians can use voice-to-text software integrated with AI to generate clinical notes (AI scribes), write referral letters, order tests, and manage other routine tasks, improving efficiency without needing to sit and manually input data.

As Bertalan Mesko aptly said, "*The doctors of the future who don't use AI will be replaced by those who do.*" It's clear that gaining a foundational understanding of digital health and AI is crucial for clinicians to remain relevant in the future healthcare landscape.

Who Thrives in Digital Health?

The digital health sector is looking for professionals who are:

- Curious and Future-Focused
    - If you're someone who looks ahead and is eager to explore new frontiers, digital health might be the perfect fit.
- Creative and Open-Minded
    - Embracing new technologies requires thinking outside the box and a willingness to learn.
- Excellent Communicators
    - Much of this work involves translating between technical teams, executive leaders, and clinicians. Bridging the gap between these groups is critical for implementing technology in healthcare.
- Adaptable
    - You need to be agile and open to continuous learning, adapting to evolving technologies and roles.
- Strong in Change Management
    - Working with others to adopt new technologies and ways of working is a key part of digital health roles, especially when there's initial caution.

Where to Find Opportunities in Digital Health

There is a wide range of job opportunities available in digital health, including roles in:

- <u>Medical Technology Companies</u>: From Microsoft and Amazon to more healthcare-focused companies like Cerner and EPIC, medical practitioners can contribute by researching, designing, and implementing health technology solutions.
- <u>Health Organisations and Hospitals</u>: Many healthcare providers

employ digital health experts to manage their tech systems, from EMR rollouts to developing digital hospitals and virtual care centres. For example, the role of Chief Medical Information Officer (CMIO) is becoming more commonplace and often allows a mix of clinical and digital work.

- Startups: Many technology startups in healthcare are founded by non-medical professionals such as software engineers. These startups need clinical co-founders or advisors to validate their ideas and ensure they are clinically sound. Opportunities for clinicians in startups can range from part-time advisory roles to co-founder positions.

Networking and Learning

Networking is one of the most effective ways to land a job in digital health. Engaging with digital health communities and following key organisations on platforms like LinkedIn can help you stay updated on job opportunities. Some important groups to follow include:

- Talking Health Tech
- AIDH (Australian Institute of Digital Health)
- The Australian Digital Health Agency
- Digital Health CRC
- CICALab (Australian Medical Angels)

Attending events and engaging with Creative Careers in Medicine can further expand your network. Many digital health roles aren't advertised in the traditional way, so connecting with industry professionals is essential.

Expanding Your Portfolio

Working in digital health doesn't require giving up your clinical career entirely. In fact, many professionals find great satisfaction in developing a portfolio career, blending clinical work with digital health roles. You may start with a part-time position in digital health and gradually transition as you build expertise in this space.

Next Steps

If you're ready to explore a career in digital health further, consider setting up a one-on-one consultation with Medical Career Planning or Creative Careers in Medicine. These organisations can help you tailor your career journey in this evolving sector.

INSURANCE SECTOR

The insurance sector offers a wide range of non-clinical roles that doctors can explore, from private health insurers to medical indemnity organisations. However, because this field is so vast, there is no single pathway into the industry. Doctors interested in working in this area should be prepared to research various organisations and understand their hiring processes and recruitment cycles.

Exploring the Insurance Sector

There are several types of insurance organisations that commonly employ doctors, including:

- Private health insurers
- Medical indemnity organisations (Medical Defence Organisations)
- Travel insurance companies and Medical Assistance companies
- Life and income protection insurers
- Government agencies like the Department of Veteran Affairs (DVA) and organisations dealing with disability assessments.

Many of these organisations hire doctors to provide expert advice or opinions for claims or insurance-related medical-legal matters. Some doctors are hired as full-time or part-time employees, while others work on a contractual, ad hoc basis, depending on the needs of the organisation.

Types of Roles in Insurance

Doctors can work in a range of capacities within the insurance industry, including:

- Medical Advisors
    - Doctors providing clinical guidance or expert opinions on claims and medico-legal issues.

- Claims Officers
    - Reviewing and processing claims by assessing medical information and summarising key details.
- Project Development, Strategic, or Management Roles
    - Working at the executive level to provide clinical oversight or lead projects related to healthcare risk management and quality governance.
- Chief Medical Officers
    - Leadership role managing other staff and assisting with escalations, governance, stakeholder management and strategy

Additionally, private health insurers are increasingly moving into the preventative healthcare space, where they require doctors to help design and manage risk reduction strategies for their clients. Doctors in these roles often focus on risk management, quality and safety strategies, or serve as medical advisors in clinical governance capacities.

Finding Opportunities in Insurance

Because insurance companies often have large umbrella organisations with smaller divisions and subcontractors, identifying where to apply can be complex. You may find opportunities in related areas such as immigration health assessments, defence health, disability assessments, or aged care medicals. The key is to decide which specific field within insurance interests you the most. It is also worth finding someone who is already working for that organisation and connecting with them, to get advice on how to find an opportunity when it does arise. You can often do this through networks like LinkedIn.

The Recruitment Process

Many insurance companies follow a structured recruitment cycle, meaning that roles may only be advertised once or twice a year. For instance, some medical-legal organisations offer internship-style positions for doctors new to the field. These companies may recruit once annually and missing the recruitment window could mean waiting another year for the next opportunity.

Therefore, it is essential to be aware of these cycles and proactively monitor job openings. The best ways to do this include:

- Online job platforms such as SEEK, JORA, or Indeed
- LinkedIn, where many companies post job openings
- Insurance company websites where you can often sign up for job alerts

Additionally, reaching out directly to HR departments at the companies you're interested in working with can help you learn about their recruitment cycles and what they look for in candidates. This proactive approach not only provides valuable information but also helps you establish contacts within the industry.

Skills Required in Insurance Roles

The insurance sector requires doctors with a solid foundation of clinical knowledge, but certain roles also require specific non-clinical skills. For instance:

- Written communication is key, as many roles involve writing detailed reports and appraising large volumes of medical documents.
- Appraisal and Analysis skills are important for reviewing medical records, pathology reports, and other clinical documentation and condensing them into relevant summaries.
- Expertise in specific medical fields is often required, particularly for medical-legal work, where doctors may need specialist qualifications or legal training.

In some cases, companies expect doctors to have additional qualifications, such as medico-legal experience or formal legal training. However, some medico-legal organisations do offer internship positions to help doctors develop these skills on the job.

MANAGEMENT CONSULTANCY

Management consulting involves helping organisations improve their performance, through optimisation or new strategies. Consultants are often called upon to provide strategic advice and insights to help organisations overcome challenges or develop specialist skills that they may be lacking. Organisations from various sectors, including public health services and private businesses, seek the expertise of management consultants.

Key Responsibilities

As a management consultant, your role includes the following tasks:

- In-depth analysis
    - You will need to fully understand the organisation by interviewing employees, gathering data, and conducting thorough analyses.
- Research & trends
    - It will be important to research industry trends, which might involve financial modelling or reviewing specialised literature.
- Data analysis & recommendations
    - Analyse data to develop business proposals that can be presented to key executives.
- Strategic advising
    - Your goal is to provide strategic recommendations, persuading key stakeholders to implement the strategies you propose.
- Problem-solving & process improvement
    - You will assess strengths and weaknesses within the organisation, providing solutions for improvement.
- Organisational change management
    - This could involve restructuring teams, technology implementation, coaching development, or strategy

formulation.

Skills Required

The following skills are essential for success in management consulting:

- Complex problem-solving

Strong communication, particularly with stakeholders

- Critical analysis
- Team collaboration

Consultants often work at a high-level, focused on strategic thinking and solving complex problems on a system-wide scale.

Work Settings and Variety

Management consultants work in diverse settings, from small medical practices to large government departments. Example tasks could range from implementing a new IT system to advising federal health departments on how to manage pandemics. The scope of the projects offers great variety and interesting challenges.

Pathways to Enter Management Consulting

There isn't a set, linear pathway to becoming a management consultant. Unlike other professions, there is no "management consulting" degree. However, several fields of study can lead to a career in this area:

- Degrees in finance, IT, marketing, business, engineering, and medicine are all viable pathways.
- Experience in the healthcare system is valued, as it gives you insights into real-world problems and allows you to offer a more nuanced perspective.

Job Opportunities

Job openings for management consulting can be found through:

- Websites of the consulting firms themselves
- Platforms like LinkedIn, Seek, Indeed, and Jora

Many firms conduct annual recruitment drives, particularly for junior positions such as analyst roles, so be mindful of application deadlines. For more experienced professionals, higher-level roles (e.g., advisor or subject matter expert) might not align with these annual cycles and can be applied for directly.

Prominent Consulting Firms

Management consulting offers opportunities at various types of firms:

- Large (top tier) international firms: McKinsey, Boston Consulting Group (BCG), Bain & Company
- Accounting firms with consulting arms: PwC, Deloitte, EY, KPMG
- Boutique firms specialising in healthcare or specific problem areas: Nous Group, Accenture, and others

When considering where to apply, be aware of the firm's specialisations and whether it aligns with your interests.

Work Environment and Challenges

The work can be demanding, with long hours, frequent travel, and tight deadlines. For individuals seeking a less stressful career after working in medicine, working at a high-level management consulting firm may not significantly reduce stress, but it offers a different type of challenge—focused on problem-solving and system-wide issues instead of direct patient care.

Setting Up Your Own Consulting Firm

For professionals with specific expertise, there's also the option to establish your own consulting firm or work as a freelancer. You can specialise in areas like digital health, build a network, and work independently with clients. Some consultants work solo or with small teams, managing everything from client acquisition to project delivery.

Professional Development

Larger consulting firms often invest heavily in your ongoing education and professional development, offering opportunities like mini-MBAs or courses through the Australian Institute of Company Directors (AICD). These firms encourage growth, skill development, and help build international networks.

Summary

Management consulting is an excellent career for those who enjoy diversity, big problem-solving, strategic thinking, and organisational development. The industry offers flexibility, variety, and plenty of opportunities for growth, whether you join a large firm or start your own.

For personalised advice or more information about pursuing a career in management consulting, feel free to reach out to Medical Career Planning or Creative Careers in Medicine. We're happy to guide you further on your career journey.

MEDICAL ADVISORS

This chapter will explore what it means to be a medical advisor, the diversity of opportunities available in this area, and how you can prepare yourself to enter this field.

What is a Medical Advisor?

The term medical advisor is quite broad and encompasses anyone who provides expert advice, analysis, and insights to health-focused or non-health-focused businesses, companies, governments or organisations. As a medical advisor, your role can vary widely based on the needs of the organisation you're working with. You may be advising on specific therapeutic areas, guiding health-related protocols or policies, or helping design safety systems.

Key Responsibilities

- Research
    - As a medical advisor, you'll spend a significant amount of time conducting research about your field and keeping up with developments in your area of expertise.
- Translation of Information
    - Your role often involves translating complex medical concepts into terms that are easily understood by non-medical stakeholders. For example, if you work for a health insurer, you'll need to explain the clinical implications of medical decisions in a way that makes sense to their financial model.
- Providing Objective, Evidence-Based Advice
    - You are expected to offer objective advice based on thorough research and evidence. This advice can help shape major decisions within the organisation, from policy development to commercial strategies.

- Problem Solving and Communication
  - Your job is to help solve complex problems in a way that doesn't compromise clinical safety, often in sectors like insurance, pharmaceuticals, or aviation, among others.
- Advising at a Systems Level
  - Medical advisors work at a macro level. Instead of focusing on individual patients, you're tasked with advising organisations, often guiding them in making large-scale decisions that could impact many people.

Skills Required

- Integrity and Objectivity: Your role is to provide independent and reliable advice that aligns with the organisation's goals, but you also need to advocate for patient safety or healthcare-related impacts.
- Communication Skills: You must be able to effectively convey medical concepts to non-medical professionals within the organisation.
- Problem Solving: Frequently, you will be tasked with solving complex problems that require in-depth analysis and creative thinking.
- Adaptability: You need to be able to work across different industries (depending on the role and organisation), ranging from pharmaceuticals to aviation, insurance, mining, or technology.

Diverse Opportunities

Medical advisors work in various industries, including:

- Pharmaceutical Companies
- Health and General Insurers
- Technology Companies
- Mining and Aviation
- Medical Indemnity Organisations
- Education and Training Organisations
- Governments

As you can see, the scope of industries that employ medical advisors is vast, providing diverse career paths depending on your interest and expertise.

How to Prepare for a Medical Advisor Role

- Medical Expertise: You don't necessarily need extra qualifications beyond your medical degree to become a medical advisor. However, having advisory experience or completing leadership and commercial courses can be beneficial.
- Upskilling in Specific Areas: Depending on the sector you work in, you

may wish to upskill. For example, if you're entering the pharmaceutical sector, additional education in pharmacology could be helpful. In insurance, financial acumen might be valuable, while in aviation, gaining some background in aviation medicine could be advantageous.

Finding Medical Advisor Roles

- Job Platforms: Medical advisor roles are advertised on platforms like LinkedIn, SEEK, Jora, and Indeed. Make sure to have a polished LinkedIn profile and follow companies of interest to stay updated on job openings.
- Networking: Connect with people already working in medical advisory roles and explore how they got into those positions. Often, networking can help you discover roles that aren't widely advertised.
- Company Websites: Many companies list job opportunities on their websites, so it's worth regularly checking these for medical advisory roles.

Pay and Negotiation

Pay in medical advisory roles can vary widely depending on experience and the size of the organisation. Unlike working in public hospitals, where pay is set by award rates, medical advisor salaries are more negotiable. You may even encounter performance bonuses or equity-based incentives in some companies. It is also possible to negotiate non salary incentives as part of your package, such as asking the organisation to pay for professional development, for example, paying for you to do a course like an MBA or paying for an executive coach. Startups, for example, may offer shares or equity or other forms of compensation instead of traditional pay structures.

Conclusion

Medical advisory roles offer a flexible and diverse career path for doctors looking to move into a non-clinical space. These roles allow you to leverage your medical expertise while working in various industries, solving large-scale problems. The diversity of roles, from pharmaceuticals to insurance or even aviation, provides excellent opportunities to broaden your horizons.

MEDICAL MEDIA

For healthcare professionals interested in media work, the opportunities are vast and varied. Media work can range from unpaid blogs and podcasts to becoming a celebrity doctor on TV or Social Media platforms. While some medical media roles are high-profile, many others are done behind the scenes. Whether you're interested in health promotion, education, or simply reaching a broader audience, the medical media world offers something for every healthcare professional.

The Value of Communication Skills in Media

Doctors naturally develop excellent communication skills through their daily interactions with patients, simplifying complex medical jargon into easy-to-understand language. Media work builds on this skill by broadening your reach. Imagine taking what you do with one patient and applying it to educate or promote health to a larger population. That's essentially what media work is all about.

The Wide Range of Media Opportunities

The spectrum of media opportunities is vast. It's important to reflect on your interests, the skills you bring to the table, and your long-term goals. Here are some examples of where you might fit in the media landscape:

- Mainstream Media: Notable examples include Dr. Norman Swan or Dr. Ginni Mansberg. These doctors often appear on TV or radio, discussing health topics for a general audience.
- Medical Journalism: This could involve writing for medical journals, blogs, or mainstream news outlets.
- Medical Spokesperson: Being the voice for health-related issues in the news or acting as a media advisor on breaking medical topics.
- Medical Advisor for TV/Film: Assisting in making sure medical aspects of TV shows or films are accurate.
- Social Media Influencer: Establishing a presence on platforms like Instagram, TikTok, or LinkedIn to share expertise and engage with audiences.

- Podcasting or Blogging: Sharing your medical expertise through digital content creation.

Many healthcare professionals engage in media work as a side project, often alongside their clinical roles. For a select few, media work can become a full-time career, but for most, it's a way to generate extra income or support their existing practice through increased visibility.

The Financial Reality of Media Work

While some media work is paid, much of it, especially in the beginning, is unpaid. This can include writing articles for newspapers, appearing in TV interviews, or offering expert opinions in news segments. Although these engagements might not offer direct financial reward, they help to build your public profile. Over time, a well-established media portfolio can open doors to paid opportunities.

Key Skills for Success in Medical Media

You don't need to be a specialist or hold a fellowship to break into medical media, but you do need strong communication skills and a passion for health education. Doctors have a unique advantage, given their medical expertise, but success in media also requires:

- Clear Communication: Being able to express your ideas concisely and in a way that is accessible to a general audience.
- Self-Confidence: Media work can be competitive, and you need to back yourself, even when faced with rejection or criticism.
- Thick Skin: Particularly in social media, doctors may face negative feedback or trolling. Being able to withstand this and continue your work is key.
- Expertise in Your Field: While you don't need to know everything, it's important to focus on topics you're passionate about and familiar with, as this will build your credibility and confidence.

The Importance of Networking

In medical media, networking is everything. Most media roles are not advertised, so you'll need to make connections in the industry. Putting yourself out there—whether through blogging, podcasting, or social media—can lead to opportunities. For example, you might be contacted to write an article or appear on a panel after someone notices your online presence.

The Importance of Flexibility

Media work often requires a quick turnaround. Opportunities may arise with little notice, such as being invited for a morning TV show. If you have a packed clinical schedule, this can be challenging. Being flexible and freeing up time for media engagements can help you stay open to these opportunities.

Building a Media Presence

If you're interested in medical journalism, starting with opinion pieces for local or national publications is a good first step. Early critiques will help you hone your writing skills and avoid bigger mistakes down the line.

For those considering social media, building a brand is crucial. Many doctors find this uncomfortable at first, but it's an essential step in establishing credibility and reaching a larger audience. A well-crafted LinkedIn profile can serve as the foundation for your personal brand.

Getting Your Foot in the Door

Roles like being a medical advisor for TV shows are rare and often go to a select group of people with connections. However, you can still network your way into these circles by joining doctor groups on social media and connecting with those already working in media.

You can also sign up for services like Sourcebottle, which seeks out expert opinions for media articles. These engagements might not be paid, but they help build your profile.

Formal Training and Further Development

While formal training isn't essential, it can be beneficial. There are organisations that offer media courses for healthcare professionals, and public speaking courses can help you improve your communication skills. Both can strengthen your confidence and abilities in the media world.

Media work can be a rewarding extension of your medical career, providing you with new ways to promote health and education. Whether it's a blog post, a podcast, or a guest appearance on TV, the key is to start and stay consistent. Most doctors in media didn't begin with major roles—they worked their way up by taking on smaller, often unpaid, opportunities.

MEDICAL WRITING

Medical writing offers a broad range of opportunities, and many healthcare professionals' express interest in this field. It encompasses a variety of writing types, from creating scientific documents to contributing to educational and promotional literature. These documents may include regulatory reports, disease or drug-related materials, research publications, journal articles, and healthcare content for websites, news articles, or even textbooks.

The key to successful medical writing is understanding your audience. Whether you're writing for patients, healthcare professionals, or regulators, it's essential to tailor your content to the level of understanding of the target reader. Developing this skill allows you to communicate effectively across different platforms and audiences.

Medical writing is not limited to clinical topics. Some doctors who enjoy medical writing also have a passion for creative writing and may publish non-medical books or novels.

Types of Medical Writing

- **Medical Journalism:** Reporting medical news for magazines, newspapers, online platforms, or social media. This often overlaps with medical media roles.
- **Medical Education:** Writing educational content, including textbooks, manuals, exam questions, and patient education materials, either for healthcare professionals or the general public.
- **Medical Marketing:** Creating promotional content for products like drugs or devices. This requires careful attention to legal advertising regulations.
- **Publications & Research:** Writing research papers, safety documents, and policies, such as protocols and medicine package inserts.
- **Safety Documents:** Involves writing policies, protocols, and patient safety information.

Each of these areas demands slightly different expertise, and it's important to continuously hone your skills to succeed.

Getting Started in Medical Writing

Opportunities in medical writing are not always advertised, and roles may not be limited to doctors. Often, these roles may have low entry-level pay. Medical journalism roles, such as editor or writer positions, are sometimes advertised on general job platforms, so it's worth keeping an eye out for them.

To build a career in medical writing, start by creating a portfolio of your work. You can do this by:

- Publishing blog posts.
- Writing articles on LinkedIn or submitting them to medical or non-medical media outlets.
- Engaging with pharmaceutical companies in roles that require writing for patient safety or regulatory purposes.
- Seeking out policy writing roles in public health at federal or state government levels.

Building a portfolio will help you demonstrate your expertise and writing skills, making it easier to land competitive roles in this field.

Writing a Book

If you're interested in writing a book, this path is rarely advertised. However, many members of the Creative Careers in Medicine community have written and published both medical and non-medical books. Reaching out to those with experience can provide valuable insight into the process, from finding a publisher to working with editors.

If you're eager to get started in medical writing, begin by producing content and showcasing your skills. As you develop your body of work, more opportunities will arise. Remember to network with others in the industry, as this is often a key to landing roles.

PHARMACEUTICAL INDUSTRY

Jobs in the Pharmaceutical Industry

The pharmaceutical industry is a dynamic field focused on researching, developing, marketing, and distributing drugs and other therapeutics. While traditionally centered on medications, pharmaceutical roles now extend far beyond drug development, offering a wide range of career paths for medical professionals.

Doctors often start in research, where you could work as a clinical research doctor, overseeing clinical trials, managing participant consent, and ensuring protocol compliance. Research positions may be found in clinical pharmacology, pharmacovigilance, or by serving as a Medical Science Liaison (MSL), medical advisor, or working in medical affairs or medicine safety.

Diverse Roles in the Pharmaceutical Industry

- **Clinical Research:** Managing trials and ensuring proper procedures are followed.
- **Medical Affairs & Safety:** Overseeing the safety and regulatory compliance of medicines.
- **Pharmacovigilance:** Monitoring drug safety and handling adverse event reporting.
- **Regulatory Affairs:** Collaborating with organisations and regulators like the Therapeutic Goods Administration (TGA) to ensure that drugs comply with legal and safety standards.

In Australia, there's no formal linear pathway into the pharmaceutical industry, but you can enter the field through various routes. Some roles require a medical degree or a PhD, while others are open to individuals with research or advisory experience.

To enter the industry, building relevant experience is crucial. A great starting point is working on clinical trials for Contract Research Organisations (CROs) or within research institutions. Experience in leadership or non-clinical advisory roles can also be beneficial.

Job hunting in the Pharmaceutical Industry

Many roles in the pharmaceutical industry aren't overtly advertised, so networking is essential. Following pharmaceutical companies on LinkedIn and signing up for job alerts are effective strategies. Even if you don't meet all the listed qualifications, it's worth reaching out, as many companies are open to upskilling promising candidates.

To gain insights, connect with industry professionals through networks like Creative Careers in Medicine or APPA (Australian Pharmaceutical Professionals Association). Engaging with pharmaceutical recruiters and building your network will help you find the right entry point for your skill set.

Why Consider a Career in the Pharmaceutical Industry?

The pharmaceutical industry offers the opportunity to work in a dynamic, intellectually stimulating environment where you collaborate with diverse teams, including those without medical backgrounds. The sector is rapidly evolving, expanding into areas like digital therapeutics, data utilisation, and holistic patient care, providing exciting opportunities for innovation.

If you value work-life balance, the pharmaceutical industry may offer better conditions compared to clinical roles, while still offering competitive salaries. Plus, you'll continually learn about new therapeutic areas and emerging technologies.

Whether you're early in your career or seeking a transition later, the pharmaceutical industry offers diverse career paths and the chance to make a meaningful impact on healthcare.

For personalised advice on entering the pharmaceutical industry, you can reach out to Medical Career Planning or Creative Careers in Medicine to schedule a one-on-one session with an expert.

PORTFOLIO CAREERS

Portfolio careers have become increasingly popular, particularly in the medical field. But how can they work in a non-clinical setting?

A portfolio career is a work arrangement where instead of having one main job, you diversify your income through several part-time roles. It allows you to move away from working for one employer and gives you the freedom to have multiple employers, essentially working for yourself. This kind of setup can also be ideal for those seeking flexibility, as many portfolio jobs can be done remotely, unlike traditional full-time roles.

Why Consider a Portfolio Career?

One of the main benefits of a portfolio career is that it breaks the monotony of doing the same job every day. You can have different interests and opportunities, adjusting them as your interests evolve. For instance, one week you may focus on teaching, while the next week, you may work on medical advisory roles.

If you're considering transitioning to a non-clinical career, starting with a portfolio approach can ease the fear of stepping away from clinical work. For example, you could reduce your clinical hours to four days per week and use the extra day to explore non-clinical roles such as teaching, medical advisory work, or tutoring. Over time, you could balance your week with two days of clinical work, one day of teaching, one day of advisory work, and maybe even a day off.

Building Flexibility and Financial Security

A portfolio career offers flexibility and independence. You can choose the roles that interest you and gradually phase out those that no longer align with your passions. It also allows you to diversify your income streams. However, it's crucial to calculate the minimum income you need to sustain your lifestyle and ensure that your part-time roles collectively meet that requirement.

Another advantage is that you can try out different roles without fully committing to them. For instance, if you give up a clinical day to try advisory work but later realise it's not for you, you can easily return to more clinical work. This approach provides the safety net of maintaining your main role while exploring new opportunities.

Networking is Key

For non-clinical portfolio careers, many opportunities come from networking rather than formal job advertisements. If you're looking for a one-day-per-week advisory role, it's essential to be proactive. Building a strong LinkedIn presence, keeping your CV updated, and connecting with potential employers are vital. Many portfolio roles are not advertised, so you need to tap into your network to discover these opportunities.

Getting Started

If you're considering a portfolio career, start by building your networks, working on roles that interest you, and understanding your financial needs. It's a great way to explore non-clinical careers while keeping your options open and expanding your skill set.

If you have further questions about non-clinical or portfolio careers, feel free to reach out to Medical Career Planning or Creative Careers in Medicine.

PUBLIC HEALTH

Public health physicians typically concentrate on specific diseases or health conditions that are more prevalent within certain communities or cohorts. For example, if you work in an area that experiences a high incidence of diseases like dengue fever, Ross River virus, or malaria, your focus might centre around these public health issues. Understanding which conditions are more common in specific regions can help you choose where to work or specialise, making public health a field where you can really focus on specific areas of interest.

The core of public health work is about advocating preventative measures and launching health campaigns to improve community-wide health. While a large portion of the role involves health promotion, there are many other aspects as well. This could include research and data analysis to identify at-risk populations or factors contributing to illness. Public health physicians are often tasked with designing and delivering health campaigns, developing public health guidelines, and providing expert advice to governments, non-governmental organisations (NGOs), or policymakers.

Public health physicians rarely work alone. They collaborate with other public health officers and health disciplines. For instance, in a campaign related to sexual health, you might work closely with sexual health physicians. Similarly, in infectious disease outbreaks, you'd work alongside infectious disease specialists, respiratory physicians, and other stakeholders, as we saw during the COVID-19 pandemic. These physicians bring expertise in epidemiology, statistical analysis, and broader public health trends to the table.

Skills and attributes of a public health physician

Key attributes for public health physicians include:

1. **Excellent communication skills** - It's vital to be able to translate complex data, research, and medical information into actionable insights that improve public health outcomes. You'll often have to present this information in a way that is easily understood by the populations you're trying to reach, as well as by non-medical stakeholders.
2. **Active listening and compromise** - Public health work frequently requires convincing populations, policymakers, or organisations to

adopt new habits or strategies. Active listening is crucial in understanding potential resistance and finding ways to create practical compromises. For instance, public health physicians had to simplify medical knowledge to influence policymakers during COVID-19.

3. **Patience and commitment to the scientific method** - Results in public health may take years to materialise. For example, the "Slip, Slop, Slap" campaign began in the 1980s, but it took a significant amount of time for it to become part of the public consciousness.

Training in public health

In Australia, public health training is managed by the Australian Faculty of Public Health Medicine, a faculty within the Royal Australian College of Physicians (RACP). The program is accredited by the Australian Medical Council. To qualify, you need:

- General medical registration.
- At least three years of postgraduate medical experience.
- A Master of Public Health (MPH).

When pursuing public health training, it's essential to review the latest guidelines on what constitutes the required three years of postgraduate experience. Sometimes, a PhD in public health might count toward this, but it's always best to check the current requirements.

You also need to secure an accredited advanced training position, which can be through public health units in hospitals, governments, or other accredited organisations, such as community health organisations or NGOs. If you think your current position fits the public health training curriculum, you might be able to get it accredited for your training.

Career prospects

Public health physicians have a wide range of career opportunities. After completing the training, you might work for government health departments, NGOs, non-profits, hospitals, or research institutions. Other sectors employing public health physicians include insurance, pharmaceutical companies, and even the defence forces. Public health offers considerable flexibility in terms of where and how you can work.

Next steps

If you're interested in pursuing public health, start by reviewing the accredited training positions listed by the RACP and building your networks in the field. Public health physicians are often open to sharing their experiences and offering guidance so ensure you reach out and enquire with the appropriate channels.

REGULATORY & POLICY

Regulatory and policy work is a diverse field within non-clinical medicine, encompassing areas such as health practitioner regulation, Medicare, complaints regulation, and pharmaceutical and medical device regulation. While there is no single pathway into this field, doctors with interests in management, leadership, law, medico-legal work, and public health often gravitate towards it. This chapter also explores opportunities in healthcare policy.

Key Regulatory Bodies

Several organisations oversee medical regulation in Australia, offering roles for doctors seeking non-clinical careers.

- **Australian Health Practitioner Regulation Agency (AHPRA)**

AHPRA collaborates with national healthcare boards and manages the registration of all Australian health professionals. It also oversees complaints, mandatory notifications, and professional conduct issues. AHPRA frequently advertises roles for Medical Clinical Advisors, who provide profession-specific clinician input. If you are interested in regulatory work, it is worth checking their careers page for job postings and expressions of interest.

- **Medical Board of Australia**

The Medical Board of Australia works alongside AHPRA to set registration and professional standards for doctors. It manages complaints and makes registration decisions, except in New South Wales, where the Health Care Complaints Commission (HCCC) assumes responsibility. The Medical Board offers roles for experienced clinicians, so monitoring their website for job openings is recommended.

- **Therapeutic Goods Administration (TGA)**

The Therapeutic Goods Administration (TGA) regulates therapeutic goods in Australia, ensuring that drugs, devices, and other healthcare products meet safety and quality standards. The TGA offers various roles, including technical, specialist, policy development, and compliance positions. Doctors with expertise in fields such as medical device regulation, pharmaceuticals, and healthcare software may find opportunities within the TGA. Salaries in government regulatory roles may be lower than private sector positions, but they often come with other benefits such as job stability and structured career progression.

- **Other Regulatory Organisations**

Beyond AHPRA, the Medical Board, and the TGA, doctors can work in other regulatory bodies, including:

- State-based complaints organisations, such as the HCCC in New South Wales
- Regulatory agencies in aviation (CASA) and other industries requiring medical expertise
- Medicare compliance and regulatory roles

Skills Required for Regulatory and Policy Work

Doctors who excel in regulatory and policy roles often share common skill sets:

- Analytical and Problem-Solving Skills: Regulatory work involves evaluating complex healthcare issues, enforcing policies, and contributing to decision-making processes.
- Strong Writing and Communication Skills; A significant portion of the job involves policy writing, drafting guidelines, and developing information sheets. Communicating complex medical and regulatory concepts in simple terms is crucial, particularly for non-clinical stakeholders.
- Open Disclosure and Regulatory Framework Understanding: Doctors in this field must work within structured regulatory frameworks and often engage in open disclosure processes.

Pathways into Regulatory and Policy Work

Doctors with public health backgrounds or extensive clinical experience often transition into regulatory work, bringing their subject matter expertise to areas such as medical device regulation and healthcare policy. Other pathways into the field include:

- Committee or advisory board roles, which allow doctors to contribute to regulation without full-time commitments
- Medico-legal roles, which involve assessing clinical cases and complaints
- Policy development positions, where doctors influence healthcare legislation and system-wide policies

How to Find Regulatory and Policy Roles

If regulatory or policy work interests you, there are several ways to enter the field:

- Job Platforms: Regulatory bodies frequently post job opportunities on platforms such as LinkedIn, SEEK, and government career portals.

- Networking and Professional Associations: Engaging with professional associations and networking with doctors in regulatory roles can provide valuable insights into job opportunities.
- Direct Applications: Many regulatory organisations list open positions on their official websites. Regularly checking these listings can help you identify new opportunities.

Regulatory and policy work offers doctors the opportunity to influence healthcare at a systems level without direct patient care. If you enjoy problem-solving, structured frameworks, and writing, this field provides a unique way to contribute to healthcare governance and public policy. While regulatory roles require strong analytical and communication skills, they can be rewarding careers that shape the future of healthcare in Australia.

RESEARCH

Research in medicine plays a crucial role in advancing medical knowledge, improving patient care, and developing new treatments. Many doctors, whether they are working in clinical practice or non-clinical roles, often engage in research throughout their careers. Research can vary from basic scientific research to clinical trials and population-based studies.

Why Consider a Career in Research?

- Contribution to Medical Advancements: Research allows you to contribute to medical advancements that can improve healthcare on a large scale.
- Professional Growth: Research can enhance your career, providing opportunities for teaching, leadership, and clinical innovation.
- Flexible Career Options: Research roles can be combined with clinical practice, allowing you to have a varied career with both clinical and non-clinical elements.

How to Get into Research

One of the most common questions is: *How do I get into research?* While research can seem daunting, with images of high-level academics or Nobel Prize winners, research roles exist at all levels. There are many ways to start a research career, whether you're a beginner or looking to transition to a more advanced role.

Key Research Pathways

- Clinical and Research Hybrid Roles
  Many doctors maintain clinical appointments while participating in research. These hybrid roles are common in hospitals and may be tied to a specific department or clinical specialty. Examples include:
  - Research Fellowships: After fellowship, many doctors in specialties like oncology, nephrology, and haematology take on research roles alongside their clinical work.
  - University Collaborations: Hospitals often collaborate with universities, providing doctors with research appointments as

professors or associate professors.

- University-Based Research Roles
  Whether you have a clinical fellowship or not, there are research roles at universities. These include:

- Professorial Positions
  These roles often require significant research experience and a clinical fellowship.
  - Research-Focused Academic Positions: Many universities offer research opportunities for doctors without fellowships, allowing for teaching and research responsibilities.
- Hospital Research Roles
  Hospitals offer a range of research roles that can be either clinical or non-clinical. These roles can vary widely, from more formal research consultant or registrar positions to niche roles such as:
  - Clinical Investigation Supervisors: Doctors overseeing the day-to-day running of clinical research trials or projects.
  - Research Registrar Positions: Roles specifically focused on contributing to research within a department, often done alongside clinical training.
- Private Sector Research
  There are numerous research roles in private sector organisations, which include:
  - Pharmaceutical and Medical Device Companies: Doctors are often needed to lead or oversee clinical trials, drug development, and other research initiatives.
  - Healthcare Companies: These companies may focus on technology, innovation, and research related to improving healthcare delivery. Finding these roles can be more challenging, so networking and regular job searching on platforms like LinkedIn are crucial strategies.
  - Non-Profit and Charity Research
    Non-profits and charitable organisations also conduct research, particularly in fields related to their mission. For example:
    - Cancer Research Charities: Organisations like the Melanoma Institute or Cancer Council often fund research, offering opportunities for doctors to get involved.
    - Health Advocacy Groups: Groups focusing on public health issues, like heart disease or diabetes, often run research programs.

These roles are often grant-funded, and reaching out directly to these organisations can open doors to new research opportunities.

- Self-Funded Research

Some doctors pursue self-funded research. This can come from:

- Personal Funds: You may choose to fund a research project yourself.
- Grant Applications: Securing grants from research councils, non-profit organisations, or government agencies can enable you to conduct your own research. Doctors at any stage of their career can apply for research grants, and many hospitals and universities have teams to help guide you through the process.

Entry-Level vs. Advanced Research Roles

It's important to remember that not all research roles require extensive experience. Entry-level research opportunities are available for those new to the field, and some common entry points include:

- Research Assistant Positions: These roles allow you to gain experience in the day-to-day tasks of running research projects.
- Junior Doctor Research Roles: Early-career doctors may be able to take on research as part of their training or apply for research positions at their hospital.

On the other hand, if you have more experience or a research background, you might be looking for:

- Principal Investigator Roles: Lead a research project or clinical trial, responsible for the overall design and execution of the research.
- Consultant Roles with Research Components: For more senior doctors, many hospitals offer consultant positions that include research responsibilities, allowing you to maintain both clinical and research work.

How to Find Research Opportunities

- Hospital Research Units: Your hospital's research unit or liaison office is often the best place to start when looking for research roles. They can provide information on current projects and upcoming opportunities.
- University Research Departments: Most universities have research liaison officers or coordinators who can help you explore opportunities within their academic units.
- Networking: Attending conferences, seminars, or research showcase days can help you meet key people in the field and learn about available opportunities. Be proactive—reach out to departments or organisations you're interested in.
- Job Platforms: Regularly search job platforms like LinkedIn or hospital career pages for research positions. Setting up job alerts can help you

stay informed of new opportunities.

- Contact Organisations Directly: If you're interested in a specific organisation, charity, or research field, reach out directly to ask about upcoming research opportunities.

Networking and Showcase Events

One of the best ways to get started in research is by attending research showcase days or conferences hosted by universities or hospitals. These events allow you to:

- Network with Researchers: Meet researchers in your field of interest and discuss potential projects.
- Learn About Upcoming Opportunities: Find out about projects in early stages that may be seeking contributors.
- Present Your Research: If you've already conducted some research, showcase days offer a platform to present your work and build your professional reputation.

Final Tips for Getting Started in Research

- Start Small: If you're new to research, look for entry-level roles or volunteer to assist on a project to gain experience.
- Seek Mentorship: Reach out to experienced researchers for guidance on how to enter the field.
- Explore Grant Options: Investigate grants and funding sources to help you launch your own research projects

START UPS & ENTREPRENEURS

Start-ups and entrepreneurship can be a career option for clinicians, particularly those interested in business and innovation. This path is ideal for people who identify a significant problem within healthcare and want to dedicate their careers to solving it. However, it's important to understand that founding a company or start-up is a challenging and often difficult journey, especially when it comes to the financial aspects.

While the prospect of starting your own business can be extremely rewarding, as it allows you to create your dream job, build your own organisational culture, and assemble your ideal team, it's a tough road financially unless you can secure funding early on.

Funding a Start-Up

Many clinicians fund their start-ups by continuing to work part-time in their clinical roles while dedicating other time, such as evenings or weekends, to building their business. A common example is a clinician identifying a workflow inefficiency in their practice, such as billing issues, and deciding to create a tool to streamline this process. In the beginning, the business might be self-funded or backed financially by family and friends.

Once the minimum viable product (MVP) is developed, some start-up founders turn to grants or external investors. Early-stage investment can come from angel investors, venture capital firms, or high-net-worth individuals. At this stage, clinicians might reduce their clinical workload and start paying themselves a small salary. However, others may choose to reinvest all funds into the business to accelerate growth. Financial challenges are common, but clinicians have the unique advantage of being able to support themselves through locum or part-time clinical work.

Myths About Technical Skills

One common misconception is that clinicians need to have technical skills, such as coding, to start a business, especially in technology-related fields. This is not true. Clinicians bring invaluable subject matter expertise and can partner with technical experts or hire developers. They may also seek support from a venture studio, an organisation that helps founders build businesses by providing the technical expertise needed.

Support and Resources

There are numerous programs and support systems available for clinician entrepreneurs. Incubator and accelerator programs like ANDHealth, MedTech Actuator, Health10x, CICALab and the Australian Clinical Entrepreneurship Program offer professional development and technical resources to help you grow your start-up. These programs provide valuable networks and mentorship, helping you overcome the challenges of building a business from the ground up.

Joining a Start-Up

For those who are interested in the entrepreneurial world but do not want to build a business from scratch, there are other ways to get involved. Clinicians can join start-ups as medical advisors, providing clinical insight into businesses founded by non-clinical entrepreneurs. This is an excellent way to gain exposure to the start-up world without taking on the full responsibility of a founder.

Medical advisors can contribute part-time, offering expertise in exchange for equity or options, which could be financially rewarding if the company succeeds. Many advisors eventually take on larger roles, such as Chief Medical Officer or co-founder.

Skills for the Start-Up World

Working in a start-up environment requires agility, adaptability, creativity, and strong communication skills. As the medical expert, you'll often work with non-clinical professionals, such as business and technical staff, which requires the ability to translate complex medical concepts into simpler terms. Start-ups are fast-paced and can be chaotic, but they offer an opportunity to be part of a diverse and innovative team.

Getting Involved

If you're interested in exploring the start-up world, networking is essential. Attend pitch nights, start-up events, and industry-specific networking opportunities. Reaching out directly to start-ups you admire and offering your expertise as a medical advisor is another pathway to getting involved. You can also explore online communities and organisations like Australian Medical Angels or Startmate, which connect entrepreneurs and potential advisors.

VENTURE CAPITAL

What is Venture Capital (VC)?

Venture capital is a form of early stage investing where funds are provided to startups or companies that may not yet be generating revenue or profit. These companies often need significant investment and guidance from investors to grow. Private equity, on the other hand, deals with companies that already have revenue and are profitable but require additional investment to grow further or transition ownership.

Why Healthcare Professionals?

Many venture capitalists invest in healthcare startups, including biotech and pharmaceutical companies. These ventures often require expert insights from healthcare professionals to evaluate whether a new drug, technology, or company is worth investing in. This role is often advisory, helping venture capitalists understand market needs, the value of innovations, and how these align with the future of healthcare.

Transitioning to Full-Time VC Roles

Some healthcare practitioners move from advisory roles to full-time positions in venture capital or private equity firms. It's generally easier for doctors to learn the financial and business side of VC than for investors to master the complexities of healthcare.

Career Progression in Venture Capital

Roles in venture capital typically begin with analyst positions, similar to management consulting, where you are responsible for conducting research, finding companies who are seeking funding, and conducting "due diligence" on potential investments. This involves analysing the industry, market trends, and the feasibility of a company's product or service. Over time, you can progress from analyst to associate, principal, and eventually partner.

In addition to full-time roles, doctors may also work as advisors, consultants, or even "venture partners," where they contribute to investment decisions without being fully immersed in the firm's operations.

Skills Needed for VC Roles

To succeed in venture capital, key skills include:

- Critical and systems thinking
- Understanding of business models and commercialization
- Knowledge of markets and global trends
- Forefront of technological innovation
- Ability to analyse market opportunities and perform due diligence

For healthcare-specific venture capital firms, such as those in life sciences and biotech, expertise in clinical trials, pharmaceuticals, or research can be highly beneficial. Companies like Brandon Capital and One Ventures often seek individuals with PhDs or deep expertise for their investments in drug and therapeutic development.

Venture Capital and Startups

Venture capital is closely linked to the startup ecosystem and innovation in digital health. Resources like Startmate fellowships offer opportunities to explore the startup world, with many influencers providing insights into the venture capital sector.

Private Equity

While venture capital focuses on early-stage companies, private equity deals with more established businesses, often improving operations or growing them. For instance, a private equity firm might buy a group of GP practices and require healthcare experts to assess their financial and operational health and potential for improvement. This involves performing due diligence on established companies to identify growth or operational enhancement opportunities.

Final Thoughts

Both venture capital and private equity offer intriguing paths for healthcare professionals wanting to transition away from clinical work. Whether you're interested in early-stage innovation or helping established companies grow, there are ample opportunities for professionals with a healthcare background to provide unique, invaluable insights.

.

OTHERS

There are other non-traditional roles that aren't purely 'nonclinical' but some doctors interested in non-clinical work also find work in these areas satisfying.

The purpose of this course is to thoroughly cover nonclinical careers, so the below jobs are highlighted, but if you wish for more information on these areas then you will need to do your own job search, or enrol in the 'nonclinical, non-traditional and non-fellowship' course on the Medical Career Planning website.

Here are some examples of some roles that are non-traditional and not necessarily nonclinical, but also not the traditional clinical roles;

- Aviation Medicine
- Clinical Investigator Supervisor
- Custodial Health
- Expedition and Wilderness or Evacuation medicine
- Immigrations Medicals/ Panel Physician
- Occupational Medicine (Particularly some of the non-fellowship roles)
- Some GP with special interest roles (Eg GPLO, some GP business or entrepreneurship opportunities)
- Business opportunities
- Roles in large organisations/ agencies such as the Australian Department of Health and Aged Care. There may be set roles for doctors that don't fit into any specific category but may expect a combination of all (Advisory, education, policy etc)

MAXIMISING YOUR SKILLS

In this chapter, we're going to explore the skills you already have, transferable skills you might not realise you possess, and areas where you may need to upskill. One of the most common concerns I hear from people considering a transition to the non-clinical world is, "I don't think I have the skills." This can be a huge barrier, stopping people from even contemplating such a move. But I promise, you already have a wealth of skills!

As doctors, we accumulate many skills, but we often don't realise which of them are transferable to non-clinical fields. Of course, it's also true that we may need to upskill in some areas—we can't assume that being a doctor automatically equips us for all non-clinical roles. The key to moving into a non-clinical field is understanding which skills you currently have, which of them are transferable, and what additional skills the new field requires. You also need to figure out if you already possess the skills they're looking for, and if not, how you can develop them.

Now, identifying these skills is not an easy task, but I'll guide you through a few steps and exercises that will help you uncover your existing skills and see where you might need to improve.

Step 1: Reflect on your skills

Start by examining feedback you've received—whether it's verbal, written, from colleagues, supervisors, or patients. Look at end-of-term assessment forms, performance on exams, patient compliments, or other written feedback, and try to identify recurring themes. For example, if you consistently get feedback that you're a fantastic communicator who can explain complex medical concepts in simple terms, that's a skill you can bring to the non-clinical world.

Step 2: Consider internal feedback

Don't rely solely on external feedback. You have many skills that may not have been recognised or mentioned by others. Reflect internally on the skills you believe you possess.

Step 3: Explore transferable skills

Transferable skills are those that can be applied across different industries, specialties, or fields. As a doctor, you already have a vast array of transferable skills. Think about how your medical-specific skills could be useful in non-clinical settings. For example, adaptability, negotiation, stakeholder management or problem-solving are highly valuable in many industries.

Step 4: Focus on teamwork

Teamwork is a skill that nearly every doctor possesses, but it's often a broad, generic term. Instead of just saying you're good at teamwork, dive deeper. What kind of teamwork are you specifically skilled at? Are you great at multidisciplinary teamwork, leading a team, delegating or co-ordinating or collaborating with others? The more specific you can be, the better.

Step 5: Create a skills quadrant

Now, let's do an exercise to help you better understand your skills using the **skills quadrant**. This will help you categorise your skills into four zones:

1. Flow skills – These are skills you're highly competent in and that also motivate you. This is your sweet spot where you feel in "flow" and are at your best.
2. Training skills – These are skills you enjoy but need to improve. They motivate you, but you're not yet fully proficient. Identifying these skills is important, as they may hold you back from applying for positions where these skills are needed. However, don't let self-doubt stop you—this is where upskilling can make a big difference.
3. Burnout skills – These are skills you're highly competent in but don't enjoy. While you can still list these on your CV if they're essential for the job, be mindful that these tasks may drain your energy.
4. Exit skills – These are skills you're neither good at nor motivated to improve. If possible, avoid roles where these skills are a primary focus.

Step 6: Identify key skills for non-clinical jobs

When looking at a position description for a non-clinical job, they will list specific skills they're seeking. Compare those to your skills quadrant to see which ones you already possess. Make a list of your top five to ten transferable skills and be prepared to give examples of how you've used those skills in a clinical setting. For instance, if they're looking for strong communication skills, you could highlight how you've presented at conferences or communicated complex medical information to patients and colleagues.

Step 7: Prepare for interviews

In interviews, you may be asked about your strengths and weaknesses. This is where the skills quadrant is particularly helpful. If you're asked about areas for improvement, you can pull from your training skills quadrant and explain what you're doing to develop that skill.

Final tip: Tailor your CV and cover letter

Your CV and cover letter are your opportunity to showcase your skills. Use the position description to align your skills with what the employer is looking for. If you feel uncertain about how to present your skills in a CV or cover letter, there is an online CV course through Medical Career Planning (MCP) that can guide you through the process.

Good luck! Your skills quadrant is a great starting point, and if you need further help, MCP's online course can provide additional support in identifying and showcasing your skills.

JOB SEARCHING

Job searching is one of the most important steps when transitioning into the non-clinical world. Identifying where you want to go is fantastic, but the next hurdle is securing the job. Successfully finding that next career step involves several key elements: crafting a fantastic CV, preparing for interviews, making the right connections, and crucially, being able to search for jobs in industries where you may not have any contacts or experience.

As medical professionals, we often don't have a lot of experience with active job searching or networking outside the medical world. It is common for jobs to come our way in medical settings—whether through private practice referrals or hospital recruitment cycles. You're probably familiar with your local health service's job portal, but searching for roles in other industries can feel unfamiliar, even daunting. That's okay! It's important to understand that it might take more time and effort than finding a job within the medical field, so be prepared to dedicate some energy to it.

Wherever you are in your career search, I encourage you to start researching now. Find out how the industry you're interested in recruits, because recruitment processes differ across sectors. Some industries rely on job boards, while others hire through recruitment agencies or direct networking. The good news is that you can uncover this information easily, starting with a simple online search.

One of the best ways to research job opportunities is by looking at job postings—regardless of whether you're planning to move geographically. Even if you live in Brisbane and intend to stay there, widen your search across the country or internationally. Looking beyond your location helps you understand what skills employers seek, how recruitment cycles work, and whether there are hybrid or remote opportunities. For example, a Perth-based company might be offering a work-from-home role, which you'd miss if you're only searching locally.

Where to start

You're likely familiar with platforms like Seek, Indeed, and Jora. These are fantastic, but there's a limitation: many of these platforms expect you to search by exact job titles, which can vary greatly across industries. For example, a "medical advisor" role might be listed under something less familiar, like "chief product innovator." Be open to trying different search terms and don't get too hung up on exact titles—this will help you uncover roles that might otherwise be hidden.

LinkedIn is another powerful tool. If you don't have a LinkedIn profile, now is the time to create one. LinkedIn is brilliant for making industry connections and researching people who hold roles you're interested in. It also has a fantastic job search function that doesn't rely on exact job titles, meaning you'll find suggestions for roles based on your skills and experience. Make sure your profile is thorough, especially regarding skills and interests, because LinkedIn will use that information to suggest jobs to you.

You can also set job alerts on LinkedIn, so you're notified when relevant roles become available. Similarly, many companies have their own careers pages or portals where you can set up job alerts. If you know the companies you want to work for, reach out directly or get in touch with their HR departments to inquire about openings and recruitment cycles. Building relationships with HR departments can sometimes lead to learning about jobs before they're even posted.

Networking is another essential strategy. Attend conferences, workshops, or industry events, and join relevant LinkedIn groups. Personal connections often yield opportunities that job boards don't. And if you're targeting a specific industry, such as digital health, these interactions can be instrumental in hearing about jobs before they go public.

Finally, if you're still interested in roles within the public hospital or government systems, remember to regularly check their specific job portals, as these roles may not appear on general platforms like Seek or LinkedIn.
To sum up, your job search strategy should include:

- Common job boards like Seek, Indeed, and Jora.
- LinkedIn's search, job alerts, and networking capabilities.
- Direct contact with companies or HR departments.
- Industry-specific networking.
- Public hospital or government job portals for roles that might not be advertised elsewhere.

Take your time, research thoroughly, and make sure to review the additional tips and resources below. With persistence and the right tools, you'll be well on your way to finding your next role.

LINKEDIN

LinkedIn is an untapped market of opportunity for medical professionals! It is the exception rather than the rule for most medical students and doctors to have a LinkedIn profile, especially early in their careers - and certainly not the mainstay application portal for clinical jobs.

Creating a LinkedIn account can help you build your network and your chances of discovering new opportunities - or being discovered for new opportunities.

LinkedIn is an invaluable tool for doctors exploring non-clinical or non-traditional career opportunities. It serves as a dynamic platform for networking, professional development, and job searching, offering features that go beyond a traditional job board. LinkedIn uses algorithms to suggest tailored job opportunities based on your experience, skills, and interests, making it easier to discover roles you might not have considered otherwise. Additionally, the platform allows you to showcase your expertise through a comprehensive profile, engage with like-minded professionals in relevant fields, and gain insights into companies or industries of interest.

Setting up a profile creates a virtual resume and allows you to connect with colleagues or follow other inspiring professionals and companies. This is often the first-place non-clinical roles will be advertised. Recruiters will often approach people for roles they think they are suitable for, through LinkedIn.

While you do not need to post on LinkedIn to keep yourself open to opportunities, it is a fantastic way to establish your 'brand' and interests, as well as participate in online discussions. Simply liking, commenting on or sharing the posts of others can help create a brand or professional identity. If you wish to take it to the next level, you can share your achievements, opinions or interesting resources you come across.

This may be unfamiliar territory for many medical students or doctors, but it is a highly valuable and recommended step when entering into non-clinical roles.

A major hurdle for many medical students and doctors is uploading a headshot! Don't worry, you don't need one to get started but we highly recommend uploading one. This doesn't have to be professional, get a friend to take a picture of you in a nice top (or scrubs!) and you're good to go.

You can continue to build out your profile as you get more comfortable with the platform.

If you're looking to start your network, give the MCP and CCIM team and company pages a follow! We look forward to connecting with you.

FINAL WORDS

Now that you've come this far, it's time to ask yourself some important questions: Do you truly want to transition into a non-clinical role? If the answer is yes, the next step is to reflect on which areas have piqued your interest and how you want to structure your career.

Do you envision building a portfolio career, balancing various roles, or are you more inclined towards a full-time position in a single area? Once you've identified your preferred sector and work structure, it's time to build your network. Connecting with others in the industry can help you gain valuable insights and potential job leads.

Next, you'll want to assess whether you have all the transferable skills needed for that field or if there are gaps that you need to fill. This might involve upskilling, taking relevant courses, or gaining further education to enhance your qualifications.

Once you feel ready, the job search process begins. You should revisit the strategies we covered earlier for non-clinical job searches. But before diving into that, it's crucial to have a strong CV tailored to the non-clinical world.

If you're unsure about your CV, ask someone in the industry you're targeting to review it. A CV for non-clinical roles can be quite different from a traditional medical CV, often requiring a different structure and additional sections. If you feel like you need support in building or refining your CV, Medical Career Planning offers a specific course to guide you through crafting a non-clinical CV and cover letter.

Once your CV is in great shape, the next step might be preparing for interviews. Interviewing can be a daunting process, especially if you haven't done many in the past, as is often the case in clinical medicine. Non-clinical interviews are common in the corporate world, so it's essential to feel confident. Medical Career Planning has an online course dedicated to helping you prepare for these non-clinical interviews, offering tips and advice to boost your confidence and increase your chances of success.

Finally, I encourage you to reach out to our team if you have any further questions or need additional support. Visit our website at www.medicalcareerplanning.com.au, and be sure to check out Creative Careers in Medicine, an excellent resource available through Facebook. Best of luck with your job search in the non-clinical world, and don't hesitate to reach out for any guidance along the way!

ABOUT THE AUTHORS

Dr. Ashe Coxon is a General Practitioner, Career Development Practitioner, and the Director and Founder of Medical Career Planning, an organisation established in 2014 to support medical students, doctors, and healthcare professionals in finding career satisfaction and discovering the right career path. Dr. Coxon is passionate about helping individuals transition into fulfilling careers that align with their skills and values.

Dr Coxon has worked across many fields, clinical and non-clinical, including traditional general practice, education, administration, business ownership, occupational medicine, psychiatry CMO work, consultancy, medical writing and advocacy.

Dr. Amandeep Hansra is a General Practitioner and has worked extensively in a variety of non-clinical and leadership roles. Her career spans the corporate sector, public service, start-ups, digital health and venture capital. She has held directorships in multiple companies and is the founder of Creative Careers in Medicine, a community with over 25,000 members (As of 2025) that assists healthcare professionals in building careers outside of traditional clinical practice.

Together, Dr. Coxon and Dr. Hansra have developed this book to address the growing interest in non-clinical careers within the healthcare sector.

Made in the USA
Monee, IL
04 November 2026

67383634R00046